TOUCH

THE MOST IMPORTANT ROLE OF THE NURSE IN CARING FOR A PATIENT

Since there are some nurses out there that like you to be short and to the point about a topic I have decided to write this shorter version of "To Nurse Means to Nurture: The Need for Nurses to Comfort their Patients" to get right to the point and solely base this book on the subject of "touch" in caring for a patient. Some nurses think it is not in their job description to "touch" their patients. Some act as if they never read anything or saw anything about the subject of "touch" in their studies but I'm here to show you that it's there. I was shocked to find out for the first time in 2012 at a specialist's office I went to one time only that the nurses thought it was not in their job description to comfort their patients, especially "touch" their patients. This was an isolated incident. However, beginning in about 2014 through the first part of 2016, I ran into several other nurses, mainly ones I never saw before that came up with this very same thing, and I thought, "Where are these people getting this from?" You're not a bunch of professionals that are just taking care of a bunch of robots. You are "nurses" who are the "caretakers of people" who are human beings "that need the love and affection of those around them", "especially those taking care of them", "especially in a hospital", and "especially when having tests and invasive procedures done on them". I know you are probably thinking, "But that's not our job. We're not here to take care of a bunch of kindergartners. We shouldn't have to treat adult patients like little kids." In this book I would like to show you that "quite the opposite is true". Please read along as I quote medical professionals from various college textbooks of nursing and nurse educational materials on the subject of "touch". "I think you will find the results to be shocking". You're in for one big surprise, because "you're about to find out that nurses are in fact supposed to "touch" their patients" and "some places in these college textbooks of nursing and nurse education books even tell them to do so" when they take care of their patients no matter what is being done, but especially when they are hospitalized or having procedures.

"Touch" is one of the nurse's most potent forms of communication."

> Fundamentals of Nursing, 7th Edition, page 353, Potter and Perry, Mosby Elsevier, 2009

"In today's fast-paced technical environments, nurses are required more than ever to bring the sense of caring and human connection to their clients (see Chapter 8). "Touch" is one of the nurse's most potent forms of communication. Nurses are privileged to experience more of this "intimate form of personal contact" than almost any other professional. "Touch" conveys many messages, such as "affection", "emotional support", "encouragement", "tenderness", and "personal attention".

> Fundamentals of Nursing 7th Edition, page 354, Potter and Perry, Mosby Elsevier, 2009

"Comfort Touch" such as "holding a hand", is especially important for vulnerable clients who are experiencing severe illness with its accompanying physical and emotional losses."

> Fundamentals of Nursing 7th Edition, page 354, Potter and Perry, Mosby Elsevier, 2009

"In older persons, "touch" increases a sense of "safety", increases "self confidence", and decreases "anxiety".

> Fundamentals of Nursing 7th Edition, page 354, Potter and Perry, Mosby Elsevier, 2009

"Students may initially find giving intimate care stressful, especially when caring for clients of the opposite gender (Seed 1995). Students learn to cope with intimate contact by changing their perception of the situation."

> Fundamentals of Nursing 7th Edition, page 354, Potter and Perry, Mosby Elsevier, 2009

"Since much of what nurses do involves "touching", you need to learn to be sensitive to others' reactions to "touch" and use it wisely."

>Fundamentals of Nursing 7th Edition, page 354, Potter and Perry, Mosby Elsevier, 2009

"Touch" should be used as "gentle" or as firm as needed and delivered in a "comforting", non threatening manner."

>Fundamentals of Nursing 7th Edition, page 354, Potter and Perry, Mosby Elsevier, 2009

"The nurse uses "touch" to communicate."

>Figure 24-2, Fundamentals of Nursing, 7th Edition, page 354, Potter and Perry, Mosby Elsevier, 2009

"Nurses can use "touch" and eye contact to enhance a client's self-esteem."

>Figure 27-4, Fundamentals of Nursing, 7th Edition, page 417, Potter and Perry, Mosby Elsevier, 2009

"Caring is central to nursing practice, but it is even more important in today's hectic health care environment. The demands, pressure, and time constraints in the health care environment leave little room for caring practice, which results in nurses and other health professionals becoming cold and indifferent to client needs (Watson, 2006a). Increasing use of technological advances for rapid diagnosis and treatment often causes nurses and other health care providers to perceive the client relationship as less important. Technological advances become dangerous without a context of skillful and compassionate care. "It is time to value and embrace caring practices and expert knowledge that are the heart of competent nursing practice (Brennen and Wrubel, 1989; Lesniak, 2005)." When you engage clients in a "caring and compassionate manner", you learn that the therapeutic gain in caring makes enormous contributions to the health and well being of your clients."

"Have you ever been ill or experienced a problem requiring health care intervention? Think about that experience. Then consider the following two scenarios and select the situation that you believe most successfully demonstrates a sense of caring:

A nurse enters a client's room, greets the client "warmly" while "touching" the client "lightly on the shoulder", makes eye contact, sits down for a few minutes and asks about the client's thoughts and concerns, listens to the client's story, looks at the intravenous (IV) solution hanging in the room, briefly examines the client, and then checks the vital sign summary on the bedside computer screen before departing the room.

A second nurse enters the client's room, looks at the IV solution hanging in the room, checks the vital sign summary sheet on the bedside computer screen, and acknowledges the client but never sits down or touches the client. The nurse makes eye contact from above while the client is in the vulnerable horizontal position. The nurse asks a few brief questions about the client's symptoms and then leaves.

There is little doubt that the first scenario presents the nurse in specific acts of caring. The nurse's calm presence, parallel eye contact, attention to the client's concerns, and "physical closeness" all express a "person-centered", "comforting approach".

In contrast the second scenario is task-oriented and expresses a sense of "indifference" to the client's concerns.

During times of illness or when a person seeks the professional guidance of a nurse, caring is essential in helping the individual reach positive outcomes."
> Fundamentals of Nursing, 7th Edition, Potter and Perry, page 96, Mosby Elsevier, 2009

"As nurses deal with health and illness in their practice they grow in their ability to care. Nursing behaviors related to caring include providing presence, a "caring touch", and "listening". "Nurses" demonstrate "caring" using a caring approach in each encounter with clients."

> Fundamentals of Nursing 7th Edition, page 100, Potter and Perry, Mosby Elsevier, 2009

"Touch" is relational and leads to a connection between nurse and client. "Touch" involves contact and noncontact touch (Fredrickson, 1999). "Contact touch" involves obvious "skin-to-skin" contact, where as non contact touch refers to eye contact. It is difficult to separate the two. Both in turn are described within three categories: task oriented touch, "caring touch", and protective touch (Fredrickson, 1999)."

> Fundamentals of Nursing, 7th Edition, page 101, Potter and Perry, Mosby Elsevier, 2009

"Caring touch" is a form of nonverbal communication, which successfully influences a client's "comfort" and "security", enhances self esteem, and improves reality orientation (Boyek and Watson, 1994.) You express this in the way you "hold a client's hand", "give a back massage", "gently position a client" or participate in a conversation."

> Fundamentals of Nursing 7th Edition, page 101, Potter and Perry, Mosby Elsevier, 2009

"When using a "caring touch", the "nurse" is "making a connection with the client" and "showing acceptance of the individual" "Tommansini, 1990)."

> Fundamentals of Nursing, 7th Edition, page 101, Potter and Perry, Moby Elsevier, 2009

"Touch" is a primal need, as necessary as food, growth, or shelter. Think of "touch" as a nutrient transmitted through the skin and "skin hunger" as a form of malnutrition that has reached epidemic proportions in the United States, especially among older adults (Fontaine, 2005)

> Fundamentals of Nursing 7th Edition, page 784, Potter and Perry, Mosby Elsevier, 2009

"Older adults need "touch" as much as or more than any other age group. However, "skin hunger" or "poverty of touch" is often acute among older adults. It is an unfortunate coincidence that older adults often have fewer family members or friends to "touch" them at a time when "simple touch" could be an enhanced form of communication when other senses are reduced "Dossey and others, 2005).

> Fundamentals of Nursing, 7th Edition, Box 36-5, page 784, Potter and Perry, Mosby Elsevier, 2009

"Simple touch" helps older adult clients feel more "connected to" and "accepted" by those around them and to their environment. "Touch" enhances self-esteem and sense of worth. A nurse who reacts adversely to the skin changes of older people often finds it difficult to "touch" an older client. The nurse's reluctance then communicates a negative message to the older adult (Dossey and others, 2005)."

> Fundamentals of Nursing 7th Edition, Box 36-5, page 784, Potter and Perry, Mosby Elsevier, 2009

"The Fundamentals of Nursing Book says this about Emotional Comfort on page 347, Box 24-5.

"Recently hospitalized clients described "emotional comfort" as a pleasant positive feeling and state of relaxation that resulted from therapeutic interactions. Clients described emotional discomfort as unpleasant negative feelings and tension. Personal control over the situation contributed to emotional comfort."

"Therapeutic interactions" helped the client achieve control and were associated with "emotional comfort". Clients perceived a positive link between "emotional comfort" and recovery."

> Fundamentals of Nursing, 7th Edition, page 347, Box 24-5, Potter and Perry, Mosby Elsevier, 2009

It goes on to say the following about Application to Nursing Practice:

"Clients perceive a connection between the mind and body. Increased emotional comfort increases "physical comfort" and enhances recovery. "Nurse-clients therapeutic interactions" improve the clients emotional and "physical comfort". Using "therapeutic communication" to increase the client's perceived control of the situation and the environment increases comfort." (Williams AM, therapeutic context, Int J Nurse Study 43 (4); 405; 2006)

> Fundamentals of Nursing, 7th Edition, page 347, Box 24-5, Potter and Perry, Mosby Elsevier, 2009

In the Fundamentals of Nursing Book on page 131 you will see in Figure 10-3 that a female nurse is "holding a patient's hand" and "puts her other hand just below her shoulder on her arm" as she talks to her.

> Fundamentals of Nursing, 7th Edition, page 131, Figure 10-3, Potter and Perry, Mosby Elsevier, 2009

In Figure 25-3 on page 377 a female nurse "puts her arm on a female patient's back" when they walk them down the hall.

> Fundamentals of Nursing, 7th Edition, page 377, Figure 25-3, Potter and Perry, Mosby Elsevier 2009

In Figure 27-4 on page 417 a female nurse "touches" a male patient on the arm with her hand". The statement under this picture says, "Nurses can use "touch" and eye contact to enhance a client's self esteem."

> Fundamentals of Nursing, 7th Edition, page 417, Figure 27-4, Potter and Perry, Mosby Elsevier 2009

On page 482 in Figure 30-7 a female nurse "puts her arm around their colleague" during time of loss to support them. This is a nurse comforting a nurse. The same should go for nurses toward patients in their loss as well.

> Fundamentals of Nursing, 7th Edition, page 482, Figure 30-7, Potter and Perry, Mosby Elsevier, 2009

In the Reader's Digest: "Your Body Your Health, The Heart" there is a "friendly female nurse" on page 128 that "puts one hand under a male patient's shoulder" while checking his heart with a stethoscope with the other hand.

> Reader's Digest: "Your Body Your Health – The Heart", page 128, Reader's Digest Association, London, 2002

On page 131 of "Your Body, Your Health, The Heart" there is a female nurse "putting her arms around the arm of a male patient" to help him walk forward. She seems to be guiding him along so he won't fall."

> Reader's Digest: "Your Body Your Health – The Heart", page 131, Reader's Digest Association, London, 2002

"The caring model involves a "closeness", "commitment", and involvement in the nurse-client relationship."

> Fundamentals of Nursing, 7th Edition, page 98, Box 8-2, Potter and Perry, Mosby Elsevier 2009

Here are some comments from the story, "The Power of Touch" from AARP magazine on the importance of touch in the field of nursing.

"The Hebrew Home has put an unusual emphasis on the power of "touch" and "touch therapy". Beverly Herzog has been widowed for 21 years but she still can't get used to this absence. She bought a baby pillow which helps a little but it's not the same. 'I like being touched, being stroked, being held', says Herzog, who lives in the Hebrew Home at Riverdale, a skilled nursing facility in New York. 'Anyone who says they don't isn't telling the truth. You feel abandoned if you haven't been touched. We all need somebody." said Herzog." (Page 38)
> The Power of Touch, pages 37-43, AARP Magazine,
> December 2015-2016

"The Hebrew Home has put an unusual emphasis on that idea. The staff here is encouraged to "hold resident's hands" and "offer gentle caresses". Beauticians are trained to massage the feet during pedicures, as well as the scalp and neck during shampoos. And, intimate relationships between residents are not discouraged – a rarity in long term care."
> The Power of Touch, pages 37-43, AARP Magazine,
> December 2015-January 2016

"Herzog has taken full advantage of this ground breaking policy."
> The Power of Touch, pages 37-43, AARP Magazine,
> December 2015-January 2016

"When you're younger, it might be easy to take "touch" for granted. Old people may loose their sense of touch, but ironically need to be able to receive touch all the more"
> The Power of Touch, pages 37-43, AARP Magazine,
> December 2015-2016

"Depriving newborns of "touch" is disaster" – growth is slowed, and serious cognitive and behavioral disorders emerge that can persist into adulthood. "Touch" is crucial for forgoing the first emotional bond with a parent and for creating the unique human experience."

> The Power of Touch, pages 37-43, AARP Magazine, December 2015-2016

"Seeing believes", wrote the 18th century English Physician Thomas Fuller, "but Feeling's the truth."

> The Power of Touch, pages 37-43, AARP Magazine, December 2015-January 2016

"Doctors who "touch" their patients are not only considered more caring – their patients have better outcomes."

> The Power of Touch, pages 37-43, AARP Magazine, December 2015-January 2016

"Therapeutic Touch" lowers levels of the stress hormone Cortisol and increases the amount of Oxytocin, the so called love hormone, which is credited with mother-and-child bonding, among other things. When we put our hands on each other, we're tapping into deep associations between "touch" and emotion that are kind lit at the dawn of life."

> The Power of Touch, pages 37-43, AARP Magazine, December 2015-January 2016

This place did more for their residents than I am asking of you. I'm just asking for hugs (putting my right ear on your cheek) from chipper acting, cheery female nurses with motherly personalities when I need to and for you to rub my head to calm me down and hold my hand during needle sticks and I feel like I am being scolded for asking.

"A surrogate – is a substitute figure, especially a person of authority, who replaces a father or mother in one's feelings."
> Webster's New World Dictionary, 2nd Edition, David B. Garualive, Editor in Chief, William Collins + World Publishing Company, Incorporated, 1976

"Combining medical technology and the "human touch", health care workers administer care around the clock, responding to the "needs" of millions of people – from newborns to the critically ill."
> Health Care, The Big Picture, Chapter 1, Page 1, Video Number 1, Health Care Career Vision Book and DVD, JIST Works, America's Career Publisher, The Editors @ JIST, JIST Publishing 2008

"Along with the long list of duties EMTs and Paramedics are given this is included in the list, "comfort" and "reassure patients.""
> Health Care Career Vision Book and DVD, page 384, JIST Works, America's Career Publisher, The Editors @ JIST, JIST Publishing, 2008

"Here is what the Health Care Career Vision Book has to say about Licensed Practical and Licensed Vocational Nurses:

"Care for ill, injured, or "disabled people" in hospitals, nursing homes, clinics, private homes, group homes, and similar situations."
> Quick Look, page 88, Healthy Care Career Vision Book and DVD, America's Career Publisher, The Editors @ JIST, JIST Publishing, 2008

"Registered Nurses are to 'administer nursing care to ill, injured, convalescent, or "disabled patients". They are to "assess: patient health problems, and "needs", develop and implement nursing care plans and maintain medical records."
> Health Care Career Vision Book and DVD, page 124, Video 39, JIST Works, America's Career Publisher, The Editors @ JIST, JIST Publishing, 2008

Here are some notes I took on the DVD videos presented on the Health Care Career Vision Book and DVD Videos:

One "female nurse" "rubbed the head of a male patient" while she and another nurse "stood on the sides of his bed." The male patient was wearing a face mask probably for anesthesia to be put to sleep for a procedure.

Another "female nurse" "held a female patient's hand".

The narrarator made this statement on the DVD.

"For all these jobs you need to be comfortable "touching" the people in your care."

Other things I noticed were as follows:

A "female nurse" "patted a lady patient on the back".

Another "female nurse" "held a male patient's hand."

A "female nurse" "put lotion on a patient's foot" and "rubbed the top of their foot" and "bottom of their leg."

The narrarator then made this statement on the DVD about Nurse Aides and Orderlies.

"You should have a desire to work with others and have compassion."

On the video about Licensed Practical Nurses I noted the following:

A "female nurse" "held a male patient's hand."

Another "female nurse" "put her hand on this male patient's shoulder".

Another "female nurse" "held another patient's hand."

The narrator made the following statement regarding massage therapists on this DVD:

"Being comfortable "touching" patients is an important necessity."

I believe he also said that many "RNs and LPNs" "give massages" as well or at least that they go into massaging during their career.

The narrarator made the following comment about Sonographers:

"Sonographers need to be willing to calm an anxious patient in a "comforting" way."

The narrator also made this statement regarding Nuclear Medicine Technologists:

"A friendly reassuring manner is almost more important than or better than expertise."

The narrator made this statement regarding Registered Nurses on the DVD:

"Registered nurses play a crucial role in providing "physical" and "emotional" care for the sick, injured, and handicapped."

The narrarator also said, "Registered Nurses have to have a strong desire to help others. You should be compassionate and the well being of patients must be completely understood and evaluated."

Here are other things I noted about the video on Registered Nurses on the DVD.

A "female RN nurse" "stroked a male patient's face."

He said, "RNs" "must make patients feel at ease before surgery."

The Narrator also said, "RNs work in Hospitals, Clinics, and Nursing Homes".

Another "female nurse" "stroked a lady patient's arm" before she went for her lab stuff to draw this lady's blood.

I noticed the following on the video about the Physician's Assistant's on this DVD:

The narrarator said, "P.A. s must be compassionate and caring when working with other people."

About surgeons the narrator said, "Surgeons must have good bedside manner."

I also noticed a "surgeon" "held a patient's hand" and "put their other hand on the patient's shoulder."

All of this was on the DVD of the "Health Care Career Vision Book and DVD". And, by the way, these weren't old, dying people either. They weren't children either. They were my age. I'm 48 years old. They were every day, middle aged people ages 30s, 40s, and 50s going for procedures and what the DVD showed the nurses do to comfort them in the same manner by the way I'm asking them to comfort me. Go see for yourself.
> Health-Care Career Vision Book and DVD, DVD Video Content, JIST Works, America's Career Publisher, The Editors at JIST Publishing, 2008

I found this statement in an AARP Magazine. Here's what it says.

"When you provide another with "comfort", when you "lend a hand", or simply "be there for someone who needs help", you transform the health of our country. Big change doesn't require a hero's effort. Just "one small act of kindness" can make you a hero to someone else. How will you participate?"

> Give Health a Hand, Medco Foundation, AARP Magazine, March & April 2010, page 67

In Funk & Wagnall's New Illustrated Encyclopedia of Family Health, 1 A-B, page 60, "a nurse" "is holding a patient's hand" while giving them anesthesia with a gas mask and "holding their stomach with their other hand."

> Funk & Wagnall's New Illustrated Encyclopedia of Family Health, 1, A-B, page 60, The Universal Standard Encyclopedia, 1958

"Dr. Diane Meier is quietly leading a revolution to treat patients (and their families too) as living, breathing, feeling individuals. And why is that so shocking?"

> AARP Magazine, September & October 2007, The Comfort Connection by Joan Kenon, pages 52, 122, and 123

"When a patient of Diane Meier, MD dies, the family receives a call or a note. "She was with me when my wife died at home", says Bert Gold of New York City still missing, Sylvia his wife of 57 years. She took me in the living room and "put her arm around me" and "started to cry". She "thanked me for letting her take care of Sylvia. Imagine."

> AARP Magazine, September & October 2007, The Comfort Connection by Joan Kenon, pages 52, 122, and 123

"Meir, 55, of the Mount Sinai School of Medicine in New York School of Medicine in New York City is one of the leading exponents of a new and growing discipline known as palliative care. "Palliative care" means soothing the symptoms of a disease, regardless of whether the patient is seeking a cure. It's a concept that's totally transforming the way doctors and hospitals treat seriously ill patients. The ideas of "easing pain" and "improving the quality of a patient's life" may seem radical, but classic medical training focuses on attacking the disease. Most doctors simply don't have time to be supersensitive Marcus Welby's checking up on patients to see how they feel. Even if they do have time, they lack the advanced training of palliative care doctors and nurses to ease symptoms such as anxiety, pain, or severe nausea. Most are better equipped to deal with microorganisms than matters of care."

    AARP Magazine, September & October 2007,
    The Comfort Connection by Joan Kenon,
     pages 52, 122, 123

I like Marcus Welby. I think nurses and doctors should be like this again.

Besides all this, these nurses may complain they don't have time to "comfort" their patients but even Gentle Annie and Clara Barton took out the time to comfort their patients in the middle of trying to catch them as they fell off of horses. Soldiers were falling left and right and Clara Barton even "cradled a soldier in her arms" when he was dying regardless of all the other soldiers around her falling, hoping she could catch them to take care of them.

You think you're busy. They were really busy and this never stopped them. They took out time to comfort their patients anyway no matter how busy they were, and that was busy if I ever saw busy. Try keeping up with that kind of pace with your patients. That's hard for me to do, and yet I would do this for them too. I just wish you would do this for me.

"Meir believes strongly that "palliative care" should not be the "death team", and she sees patients early in the course of the disease."

> AARP Magazine, September & October 2007, The Comfort Connection by Joan Kenon, pages 52, 122, and 123

"Meir is pushing for more programs and she says "too many are stuck in a medical no-where land, forced to choose between "comfort care" and "emotional support" in a hospice or a chance to keep fighting their illness."

> AARP Magazine, September & October 2007, The Comfort Connection by Joan Kenon, pages 52, 122, and 123

"Meir says, "It's not human nature to accept death and agree to give up on life. With palliative care we don't have to."

> AARP Magazine, September & October 2007, The Comfort Connection by Joan Kenon, Health Writer in Washington D.C., pages 52, 122, and 123

I have seen doctors and nurses "comfort their patients" on the St. Jude Children's Hospital Commercial several times and that includes "touching". They "hug" their patients, and "rub their heads" and "hold their hands too".

I've even seen a place on the internet I looked up where they had pictures of nurses "hugging their patients" and they had a whole slew of them.

My mother wanted me to be taken care of after she dies. She wants me to be taken care of and me be happy and have my needs met. And, even though my needs may seem unusual, my needs are my needs and that is what I need. I'm autistic and I am an Ex-Special Ed student and I have the same childlike needs I had back then.

They never went away and they never will and these needs need to be met for the rest of my life. In order for me to be taken care of, I have to be able to "get hugs" from all my church friends and from all my nurses and doctors and techs when I go to the hospital or doctor's office, and get chipper acting, cheery female nurses only who will "give me hugs" and "let me give them hugs", and "rub my head to calm me down" and "hold my hand" during needle sticks every time they are done on me. Meet my list of needs on the list, "all of them" and we are good to go. Please meet my needs.

"Lisa H. Newton in her defense of the traditional role of the nurse appeals to an argument based on the patient's needs. Because a patient may not be able to take care of himself Newton points out, 'His entire self concept of an independent human being may be threatened'…He needs "comfort", "reassurance", "someone to talk to", the person he really needs, who would be taking care of all these problems is his mother, and "the first job of the nurse is to be a "mother surrogate".

> Caring: Nurses, Women and Ethics, Helga Kuhse, page
> 58, Blackwell Publishers 1997

This is what Kaplan Nursing says about the nursing process and psychosocial integrity.

"You" utilize the nursing process cases, diagnose, plan, implement, and evaluate to promote a client's psychosocial integrity by conveying "understanding", "sensitivity", and "compassion" to a client who is experiencing stress, illness, or crisis."

> Kaplan Nursing, NCLEX-RN 2014-2015, page 186,
> Strategies and Practice and Review with Practice Test,
> Kaplan, Inc., 2014

"Nurses" "provide care" for clients who constantly interact with their environment. "Clients may have unmet needs", be unable to take care for themselves or be unable to adapt to the environment due to health problems. "You" provide "therapeutic care" so clients can adapt to their environment."

> Kaplan NCLEX-RN, Kaplan Nursing, page 186, Strategies, Practice and Review with Practice Test, Kaplin, Inc., 2014

"You" need to identify clients at risk for "sensory perceptual" alterations so you can initiate prevention measures."

> Kaplan NCLEX-RN, Kaplan Nursing, page 186, Strategies, Practice and Review with Practice Test, Kaplin, Inc., 2014

"You" should also listen attentively, "provide an atmosphere of "warmth" and trust", provide functional information as needed, and encourage clients to participate in the plan of care, promote safety and security and public education."

> Kaplan NCLEX-RN, Kaplan Nursing, page 484, Strategies, Practice and Review with Practice Test, Kaplin, Inc., 2014

"Caring- As you take the NCLEX-RN 2014 exam remember that the test is about "caring" for people, not working with high-tech equipment or analyzing lab results."

> Kaplan NCLEX-RN, Kaplan Nursing, page 11, Strategies, Practice and Review with Practice Test, Kaplin, Inc., 2014

"The first subcategory for this "client need" is "Basic Care and Comfort" which accounts for 9 percent of the questions."

> Kaplan NCLEX-RN, Kaplan Nursing, page 11, Strategies, Practice and Review with Practice Test, Kaplin, Inc., 2014

"Providing "basic care" and "comfort" for your clients is "one of your most important roles."

> Kaplan NCLEX-RN, Kaplan Nursing, page 8,
> Strategies, Practice and Review with Practice Test,
> Kaplin, Inc., 2014

"Promoting a client's "psychosocial integrity" is not just for the mental health client but for "all clients."

> Kaplan NCLEX-RN, Kaplan Nursing, page 186,
> Strategies, Practice and Review with Practice Test,
> Kaplin, Inc., 2014

"Nurses, not families, are responsible for "all" the hands on nursing care for clients in the hospital."

> Kaplan NCLEX-RN, 2014-2015 – Strategies, Practice and
> Review with Practice Test, page 186, Kaplan Inc., 2014

"Nurses" care for the whole person, not just all illness. Their focus in on "client needs;" that is how a client will respond to illness."

> Kaplan NCLEX-RN, Kaplan Nursing, page 455, Strategies,
> Practice and Review with Practice Test, Kaplin, Inc., 2014

"Nurses have to make people "comfortable" when they are "hurt" or "afraid."

> Nurses: Community Workers by Cynthia Kingeland,
> Robert B. Voyed, Compass Point Books 2003

Here are even more examples of movies about nurses in action comforting their patients:

In the movie, "Love Finds a Home" Belinda, a doctor takes care of her sister or other doctor friend when she has sharp pains and is pregnant and has a fever. Belinda put her hand on her forehead to see how hot she was. Then she pulled her blanket over her body to cover her. Then, she held her hand.

After that Belinda raised her patient's hand up and put it on the lady's face and caressed the side of the lady's face with her hand from the top of her face to the bottom of her face in a stroking motion. Belinda looked at her with deep sadness for her and was filled with compassion. Then, she stepped back and let her rest so she could sleep.

I guess some nurses don't think nurses do things like this, but they did here and I've seen several other movies where they did the same kind of thing.

In the movie, "Awakenings" a true story about patients with encephalitis, Dr. Sayre's nurse "rubs the old lady patient's head" (strokes her head) when she sees how upset she is that it is not still 1922.

Another nurse "stroked the top of the head" of the red headed lady patient "against her hair on the side of her head" and then "flung her fingers through the strands of her hair at the bottom of her head" when she tilted her head backwards to the side of the chair.

Another nurse "rubbed a lady patient's upper back" in circular motion when they looked at themselves in a mirror and said, "Are you okay?"

If you'll notice, Dr. Sayer himself even "gently touched" each of his patients as he positioned them as if to show his love for them to make them feel comforted.

On the commercial about St. Jude's Hospital on television they show various ways nurses "touch" their kid patients to "comfort" them. "I've seen them get close to them several times" and either "put their arm around them" or "put their hand on their shoulder".

It's hard to remember for sure what all I saw because I haven't seen the commercial since two weeks before I wrote "To Nurse Means to Nurture" Part I.

So, because of that, I looked up their commercial videos on the internet and loved what I saw.

On the internet video clips of St. Jude's Hospital they showed three different nurses "hugging their patients".

A male nurse was shown "hugging" their kid patient.

Then, a "female nurse" was shown "hugging" their kid patient.

Then, a toddler "ran up to their female nurse" and "their female nurse "hugged" them".

One "female nurse" "rubbed a kid patient's back."

Another "female nurse" "held a kid patient in their arms."

Another "female nurse" "let a kid patient lay their head on their shoulder".

It was wonderful. I thought it was the sweetest thing they did for their kids and it should be this way.

When I looked up nurses "comforting" patients and clicked on "Images of Nurses Comforting their Patients" "I saw a slew of pictures I had to scroll down through showing nurses doing everything for their patients I ever asked my nurses to do for me." "There was about two pages worth of these pictures".

"Several nurses" "held their patients' hands."

"Several nurses" "put their hands on their patients' shoulders."

"One nurse" was "putting their hand on their patient's back."

"Another nurse" was "putting her arm around a kid."

"The rest of these patients that were being "comforted" by "their nurses" by use of "touch" were "young to middle aged adults".

There were a few kids in between, but there must have been at least 15 or 20 pictures of young to middle aged adults in this whole slew of pictures that were "getting their hands held", "their shoulders held", and even "getting their heads rubbed".

They even showed "one nurse" "hugging a 37 year old woman."

I clicked on this picture and it went to this story about a New York Lady patient getting to reunite with her nurse who took care of her as an infant. The patient's name was Amanda Scrarpauil, and she finally got to meet the nurse that brought her "comfort" for nearly 40 years. She had a burn she was treated for as a child and she finally got to meet her nurse who took care of her as an infant and be with her again. I have a feeling from the way the rest of the story went she stuck with this nurse from there on out because she loved her so much. This was in the New York Daily Times on the internet.

Bertha got a miniature magazine last year similar to a Reader's Digest Book called "Prayer Point-Summer 2016".

On the cover of this little miniature magazine you will see a "nurse" "putting her hand on the head of a female patient" and "leaning her face down toward her" "looking at her with concern" while she is laying in a bed hooked up to an IV. This book has the title at the bottom "Life Saving Compassion".

You can't tell me nurses don't "rub their patients heads to calm them down", especially after I already saw the exact same thing on the Health Care Career Vision DVD from 2008 of them doing this for patients "my age" (not dying ones, but sick ones).

They showed "the nurses" "rub their patient's heads" too, "several times".

24

The same thing was shown on the Facing Death DVD of the patients that really were dying, but they don't have to be dying for them to do this.

These nurses do this anyway for all ages of patients when they do they're job right and don't complain it's not in their job description to do so.

When I looked up "Nurses Hugging Patients" or "Nurses Giving Patients Hugs" on the Internet and clicked on Images of Nurses Hugging patients, there were several of them, probably two pages worth of pictures of nurses hugging their patients.

When I looked up videos on nursing it was harder to find what I was looking for because they were mainly showing the technical stuff for educational purposes to show nurse students how to take a blood test or take records for example.

There was one I found from VC San Diego Medical Center, however, where two chipper acting female nurses began working with the lady patient one of these "two chipper acting female nurses "put their hands on the patient's shoulder" when they asked a question".

 Then this nurse "put her hand on her lady patient's arm" to tell her something. When she wanted to check her response ability, she told this lady, "Squeeze my hand when I say "A". The lady patient squeezed her hand. "This nurse" was "very sweet" and "had the type of personality I like in a nurse". She was "very chipper" and "sweet" and "caring." I thought it was great.

On one of these videos they had a box of words to the side that said, "To Care", "To Advocate", "To Inspire", "To Be a Nurse", "Nursing".

When I looked up a video on needle phobics, one nurse was stating, "You need to be more than careful when dealing with a needle phobic patient. They need a lot of attention." She went on to say, "When they come for me to take blood, I'm going to lay them down. I'm not going to have them sit in my chair."

This is how I have them do it. I have "a cheery female nurse lab tech" lay me down and have "one cheery female lab tech nurse rub my head to calm me down and hold my hand" while "another cheery female nurse lab tech does the blood test, shot, or IV." That's what works best for me, too.

In the Feature Films for Families movie, "Alan and Naomi" about the shy girl that got continually panicked in public especially in crowds, after a nurse took Naomi to the Mental Hospital and they showed Naomi sitting on a bench, they also showed one of the nurses "hug" one of their patients in the field and afterwards they "leaned the patient's head on their shoulder" and "gently put their hand against their head" in the front yard of the mental health hospital.

My definition of comfort has always been "to cheer up and show affection to" by talking with an uplifting spirit to your patients and "give them hugs", and "rub their head to calm them down through needle sticks" and "hold their hand", "pat them on the shoulder", and "rub their shoulder", etc.

 I've seen this my whole life as the definition of "comfort" from everyone including "parents", "friends", "teachers", "nurses", "doctors", "techs", "church friends", and "other acquaintances".

"My whole life I've seen it this way", and "now some of these nurses seem to want to redefine "comfort" as if it is something else." "Comfort to me is what it always has been", "a warm hug", "a tender touch", "a rub on the head or shoulder".

"None of this other stuff they come up with these days" is "comfort".

"It's just a lame excuse to get out of showing comfort so they don't have to get too personal with you when in reality that's what nursing is all about". It's about "mothering your patients" helping heal their wounds and "comforting them in their sorrow and pain." Even if they are not in sorrow or pain, they will be if you don't comfort them because they will feel like you don't care and they're just a number to you, and they are "starved for affection" because you didn't give it to them and their heart is broken. Is that really what you want?

"Refusing to comfort your patients" "is wrong", and any patient that comes to you "should be able to be comforted by you" if they ask you to comfort them whether you feel like it or not.

"They just need to feel loved and cared for and you are supposed to treat your patients as a mother treats her own children." "Not doing so" just causes "chaos" and "fear" and "broken heartedness" and "even if you stood a chance of saving your patient" "you may have just lost them because of what you just did." You refused them of the very thing they needed. The "comfort" "they needed" "you" "to give them," especially me. It especially causes chaos when a patient has a sensory issue in their right ear like me that can only be relieved by putting it on the cheek of the people that I like, including nurses. The disabled need this worse than ever, even more than normal people do. Not doing so traumatizes them and may cause them to lose their will to live.

They feel like me, like why bother getting well if my nurses are going to treat me like a stranger they just want to fix up and get rid of. They're just there for the paycheck and they don't care anything about me. Why doesn't anybody care?

Have you ever seen the movie, "Cipher in the Snow"? When you do this to me you are doing the same thing to me they did to this boy. This boy felt ignored by most people and felt unimportant and he felt like his emotional needs were not being met by his peers and teachers. So, am I saying this boy committed suicide? No. Watch the movie. He didn't have to.

He was so overwhelmed with emotional disappointment and sadness that when they stopped the bus on the road one day, this kid said, "Could you let me off the bus? I need to take a break."

The kid stepped off the bus and passed out in the snow and died of a broken heart. This is a true story movie.

This is what you are doing to me when you refuse to meet my emotional needs, especially when you refuse to give me hugs or let me hug you, and it has already come very close to this point in many instances.

Before 2014 I got hugs from every nurse I liked at the hospital I went to before from 2005 to 2014 and I had been in there for several procedures in Pre-Op, several x-rays or sonograms etc in Radiology, had several minor emergency ER visits (except for one or two major ones), and was an in-patient 3 times between 2005 and 2012.

Before 2014 the only people that gave me trouble about wanting a hug were one or two people in Physical Therapy, two or three people in GI, which nobody liked that department including the nurses, and once in a blue moon there would be one or two in in-patient that would not, but even that was not common.

Everyone else that was a nurse or tech in the entire hospital gave me a hug all the way from 2005 to 2014 and even in 2002 when I went then.

Before 2014 every nurse in Pre-Op would hug me, every Radiology Tech in Radiology would hug me, every Emergency Room nurse would hug me, and in most instances every In-patient nurse would hug me unless it was a day the one or two reluctant ones were working.

I even got most of the Physical Therapy people to hug me. They were not as understanding but they gave in anyway.

All the nurses in all the other departments of the hospital were happy as a lark to give me a hug.

Then, one day, I had to go to a different hospital out of my area to get a test done these people did not have.

I was even promised I'd get hugs from everyone.

 For the first time ever, with the acception of the one isolated incident I told you about in 2012 that only occurred one time where this happened, after I had trouble getting through two IV stick attempts, the nurses at that hospital began refusing to hug me after that, yelled at me for screaming through the 3rd IV stick who they had a scary lady do on me that was rough, and another girl even shoved my bed down a hallway and into a procedure room where several girls refused to hug me and made me feel panicked before they put me to sleep and if it had not been for the one girl that came in there all cheery that said, "Hello!" that I said, "Can I have a hug?" and she said, "Sure!" and her friend that came after her that gave me a hug, I probably would have got worked up into a heart attack from all the commotion.

My feelings went down after the very last girl refused to hug me but it was very shortly after that I was put to sleep.

I remember looking at the wall and then looking back at my bed trying to figure out where the two nice ones went. I was about to panic but I conked out before it got the best of me.

The very one who promised my needs would be met even snuck up behind Bertha while she was outside waiting for this to be over and said, "Mrs. Evans! What seems to be the problem here?!" Bertha said, "The problem is you promised my husband's needs would be met and they are not being met!"

The lady said, "His needs are being met! His requests are not!" There was even a security guard chasing her around and the patient advocate took this other lady's side.

A friend had come late to check on me asking if she could see me and this very same lady that gave Bertha trouble yelled at her and said, "Are you a nurse?!"

Bertha's friend said, "I don't think that's any of your business."

They left very big bruises on my arm from the IV after being stuck 4 times.

And, by the way after I screamed on the 3rd stick, I grunted on the 4th stick and the girl that was my nurse there said, "You did good! If you had not have, there's a guy standing out there that would have come in here next!"

I took that as a threat that a male IV tech was going to stick me hard if that lady couldn't get it done.

Bertha thought they may have meant the security guard, since she had problems with him later, but I never saw him and I didn't even do anything. I was just panicked in excruciating pain feeling like a victim to those that were around me.

Also, I told them I only wanted cheery female nurses doing this.

This lady that substituted to do the 3rd and 4th IV stick on me was a "very serious trended, grumpy female nurse" in her upper 50s or early 60s.

When I told most of my nurses at my local hospital this happened they felt sorry for me and thought it was terrible. They even said, "What do they mean it's not in their job description to meet your needs? They're always supposed to meet your needs."

Then, my own local hospital started hiring stoic acting nurses in inpatient and ER and all the chipper acting cheery female nurses that knew me for years in those departments of the hospital quit their jobs and went somewhere else. I didn't know what was going on with this.

Now, all of a sudden, in 2014 and 2015 they were starting to act the same way as the girls at the other hospital with this, "We're not allowed to touch anybody!" thing or "We can't touch anybody" thing and this "It's not in our job description to comfort our patients" thing, and, "We can't touch you", "We can't hug you.", or "You can't hug me. That's invading my space." thing and for the first time ever, several nurses began refusing to hug me, but most of the ones that did never really met me before that year.

I thought, "What's going on here?! What is this, "The Day of the Opposites?!"

I told a girl that was taking care of me in the Radiology department of the hospital that did still understand me what happened, but that particular girl was on a conformity kick and thought, "Well, if they're not going to meet his needs, neither am I" and then she turned the whole Radiology department against me.

Before you know it, I was told no one was going to hug me or rub my head to calm me down through a needle stick ever again.

This girl complained she was having to take care of a kindergartner and I was a man.

And, one other individual that worked there told Bertha I needed to find a Children's Hospital where I would be better understood.

She told Bertha, "The nurses at this hospital are not trained to take care of autistic adults. He needs to find another hospital he can go to where they are. Maybe a special needs hospital because the Children's Hospital may think he's too old for theirs."

That's when we went fishing for other places and a couple of them started out meeting my needs but after like two visits they did the same thing.

So that's why we finally came over here where we are now.

We knew people over here that were nurses that already understood me and things worked out much better when we did.

Not only that, I found out last year that one of the nurses in your area had friends that were bullied by the very same person and their bunch that bullied me for the test I went to at the one hospital that was mean to me and she was on my side, and she was a cheery female nurse, and she did give me hugs and rubbed my head to calm me down and held my hand for her test because she understood. I need this from now on.

Please remember to show compassion in your care and comfort your patients the way they need comforted. Thank you.

"Certain forms of "touching" behaviors indicate "affection". For example, "cheek patting", "hand patting", and "chucking under the chin" are valued forms of "affection" in North America. The "laying on of hands" is a common expression indicating curative and comfort actions. This expression is often attributed to individuals in the healing professions such as religion, medicine, or 'nursing'. Tactile contacts vary considerably among individuals, families, and cultures. Some families have a great deal of tactile contact between all members of the family. Other families, even within the same culture have minimal contact. Appropriate forms of 'touch' can be helpful in 'reinforcing caring feelings' by the 'nurse'.

> Fundamentals of Nursing: Concepts and Procedures,
> Barbara Kozier and Glenora Lea Erb, Addison-Wesley
> Publishing Company, 1979, page 407

The use of "touch" alone often says much more than words for many patients such as those who are terminally ill or who are unable to speak."

> Fundamentals of Nursing: Concepts and Procedures,
> Barbara Kozier and Glenora Lea Erb, Addison-Wesley
> Publishing Company, 1979, page 407

"Disabled persons are entitled to have their 'special needs' taken into consideration at all stages of economic and social planning."

> Fundamentals of Nursing: Concepts and Procedures,
> Barbara Kozier and Glenora Lea Erb, Addison-Wesley
> Publishing Company, 1979, page 77, Declaration on the
> Rights of Disabled Persons, #8

I am autistic and this should apply to me.

"In the Declaration on the Rights of Disabled Persons adopted by the General Assembly of the United Nations in December 1975 thirteen points are made. This declaration includes the definition of disabled '…deficiency, either congenital or not, in his or her physical or mental capabilities.'"

> Fundamentals of Nursing: Concepts and Procedures,
> Barbara Kozier and Glenora Lea Erb, Addison-Wesley
> Publishing Company, 1979, page 76, Rights of Special
> Groups"

"The American Hospital Association (AHA) approved a Patient's Bill of Rights in 1973; the United Nations adopted the Declaration of the Rights of Disabled Persons in December, 1975. Bills are being passed that provide for the rights of patients in some states and provinces."

> Fundamentals of Nursing: Concepts and Procedures, Barbara Kozier and Glenora Lea Erb, Addison-Wesley Publishing Company, 1979, page 76, Rights of Special Groups

"Since the publication of the AHA Bill, a number of other rights statements have been made public, notably for the handicapped, the dying, the retarded and the elderly."

> Fundamentals of Nursing: Concepts and Procedures, Barbara Kozier and Glenora Lea Erb, Addison-Wesley Publishing Company, 1979, page 76, Rights of Special Groups

So, these nurses are supposed to meet my "special needs" because I am disabled and I do have special needs.

"Nurses are repeatedly faced with divided responsibility. On the one hand, the nurse is frequently an employee responsible to a hospital or health agency. On the other hand, the nurse is a professional person responsible to the professional ethics of an association and the standards of the profession. Last, "the nurse is responsible to and for patients" and is "taught to respond to their needs" "in a therapeutic manner."

> Fundamentals of Nursing: Concepts and Procedures, Barbara Kozier and Glenora Lea Erb, Addison-Wesley Publishing Company, 1979, page 66

"The need for "love" is so basic that it has been described as the bony structure of man's whole emotional life (Caprio 1965:16). So much has been written on the subject of love by philosophers, poets, novelists, and behavioral scientists that the meaning of love is not always clear. To define love is difficult. There are many kinds of love, such as "mother love", romantic love, love between friends and family members and love of God.

Perhaps it is enough to understand that love is accomplished "with the heart" and "not the mind", that "love is a feeling-an acting response rather than an intellectual process". "Love" is also a strong positive feeling that is not possessive. Some characteristics of love are outlined as follows:

1. "Love" is not only a subjective feeling that a person has (an emotion) but also a series of acts by which one person conveys to another the feeling that someone is deeply involved and profoundly interested in the person and the person's welfare.

2. "Love" is unconditional; it makes no bargains but conveys that one person is concerned for another person that someone is there to give support and to contribute to the other's development as best as possible because the one values the other for what he is and as he is.

3. "Love" is supportive; it conveys to the other that you will always be present when the person most needs you, that you will neither condemn nor condone but that you will be there to offer your sympathy and understanding. Whatever the other needs as a human being she shall have. It is tolerant but not dependent (Montague 1974:15)
    Fundamentals of Nursing: Concepts and Procedures, Barbara Kozier and Glenora Lea Erb, Addison-Wesley Publishing Company, 1979, page 106, The Need for Love and Affection, Love and Belonging Needs

"The need for "love" is met in many ways. In some situations, "nurses" can become the "surrogate parents" for young children who are in the hospital by supplying them with the "affection" and the "physical closeness" they need. With adults and elderly people the role of the nurse is less concrete. However, "in all instances" and interest in the welfare of people and a caring and supportive attitude need to be communicated.

> Fundamentals of Nursing: Concepts and Procedures,
> Barbara Kozier and Glenora Lea Erb, Addison-Wesley
> Publishing Company, 1979, page 106, The Need for Love
> and Affection, Love and Belonging Needs

"These can be conveyed in many ways: by 'touching', by 'staying with a patient when a patient is frightened', and by listening and communicating in a friendly manner."

> Fundamentals of Nursing: Concepts and Procedures,
> Barbara Kozier and Glenora Lea Erb, Addison-Wesley
> Publishing Company, 1979, page 106, The Need for Love
> and Affection, Love and Belonging Needs

"A nurse" can help build trust and security with a patient by (a) being a real person herself (genuineness); (b) "caring warmly" for the patient (nonpossessive warmth); and (c) attempting to understand him accurately (accurate empathy).

> Basic Nursing: A Psychophysiologic Approach, W.B.
> Saunders Company, 1979, Sorenson, Luckman, page 39

"Nurses" are responsible for 'meeting the needs' of clients whose care involves technical equipment."

> Kaplan Nursing, Kaplan NCLEX-RN, 2014-2015,
> Strategies, Practice, and Review, page 456, Kaplan Inc.,
> 2014

"Rehabilitation begins when a patient first comes in contact with a health professional. It is not the final stage of treatment. On the contrary, rehabilitation is the underlying theme of all nursing and medical care.

> Basic Nursing: A Psychophysiologic Approach, W.B.
> Saunders Company, 1979, Sorenson, Luckman, page 241

"Rehabilitation involves assessment of the patient's physical and psychosocial needs and abilities. Both short-term and long-term assessments are necessary. A skillful nurse consistently evaluates the care she gives in relation to the previously identified, "individualized patient's needs" and "goals."

> Basic Nursing: A Psychophysiologic Approach, W.B.
> Saunders Company, 1979, Sorenson, Luckman, page 241

"Creating a "therapeutic environment" means providing circumstances within which a person can feel comfortable and can work toward health when this is possible. This involves consideration of 'physical comfort' and 'psychological comfort'."

> Basic Nursing: A Psychophysiologic Approach, W.B.
> Saunders Company, 1979, Sorenson, Luckman, page 30

"While a nurse can get great satisfaction from her work, "the helpful nurse does not allow her personal needs to take precedence over the needs of the patient". The helpful nurse is a "real person" within the nurse-patient relationship. However, the focus of the interactions is directed toward "patient need".

> Basic Nursing: A Psychophysiologic Approach, W.B.
> Saunders Company, 1979, Sorenson, Luckman, page 26

"Emotional regression" (going back to earlier stages of psychological development) may produce conflict for a patient if he realizes that although he is an adult, and thus should act as an adult, he 'wants to' or 'needs' to act in rather 'childlike ways'".

> Basic Nursing: A Psychophysiologic Approach, Sorenson
> Luckmann, W.B. Saunders Company, 1979, page 152

I need to be able to open up and be able to act like a child and be treated like a child and be allowed to say childish things and make childish requests when I am with nurses especially in the hospital setting and I need to be able to be comforted like a child because I have childlike needs. If I say something stupid at any point that a nurse might normally take wrong, I need them to look at it like, "He's just being a kid. Don't be down on him. He's just a child in a man's body acting like a child because he's socially and emotionally 5 years old whether he's an adult or not so let him be that way and don't make anything of it. He's just being a kid. Besides that he requires a lot of attention and affection because of his disability and he needs us to be like mothers to him. If he says anything strange don't take it too seriously, he's just being a kid at heart. He doesn't mean anything by it. And, if he asks us to baby him to death, just do it, he wants us to be his mothers and this is what he needs."

"At times a nurse may feel a sense of discomfort in response to what a patient is saying or the specific manner in which he is acting, however, she still strives to convey a genuine acceptance of the patient as a person. That is to say, the attitude the nurse tries to convey to the patient is: "I care about you even though these particular words or this specific behavior of yours makes me uncomfortable."

> Basic Nursing: A Psychophysiologic Approach, Sorenson Luckmann, W. B. Saunders Company, 1979, page 132

"This acceptance of the patient as a person requires that the nurse demonstrate a genuine appreciation of the patient's situation rather than only looking at this behavior by itself and reacting to it without attempting to understand what prompts the behavior."

> Basic Nursing, A Psychophysiologic Approach, Sorenson Luckmann, W. B. Saunders Company, 1979, page 132

"Another key word to understanding is "individuality". Although clinicians attempt to categorize "disabilities" and understand the psychology of each "disability", nurses cannot lose track of the unique aspects of each human being and the unique skills, past learning experiences, environmental, social and family influences that have made that individual."

>Comprehensive Rehabilitation Nursing, Nancy Martin, Nancy B. Holt, Dorothy Hicks, McGraw Hill Book Company, 1981, page 137

"The nurse's nonjudgmental acceptance of the client is an important characteristic of the relationship. Acceptance conveys a willingness to hear a message or to acknowledge feelings. It does not mean you always agree with the other person or approve of the client's decisions or actions. A helping relationship between nurse and client does not just happen – you create it with care, skill, and trust."

>Fundamentals of Nursing, 7th Edition, Potter and Perry, Mosby Elsevier, 2009, page 346

So, regardless of what a patient says or does that may seem strange to you, you are supposed to consider the individuality of the patient rather than judge them based on how you think every one else would think if they said or did the same things and accept them the way they are and continue to comfort them and console them in a way that comforts them and treat them in the same manner you always have. If they have done anything that offends you, you should try to overlook what they have said or done that may have crossed you the wrong way and be willing to forgive them of whatever they might have said or done that has offended you and go on, but still be willing to "touch" them and accept them the way they are. So, even if I do strike you strange, you need to be willing to "touch" me to "comfort me in a way that comforts me" the way you always have and leave your cross feelings you may have toward me behind. I need your comfort and compassion no matter what I say or do that may offend you and for you to always be there for me and treat me as if I was your own little child.

"In their search for security patients often hope to find in nurses the reassuring qualities of "sympathy", "tenderness", "understanding", and "gentleness" tempered with firmness. The careful reader will observe that these are qualities often attributed in the "ideal mother figure."

> Basic Nursing: A Psychophysiologic Approach, Sorenson Luckmann, W.B. Saunders Company, 1979, page 152

"The patient thus often looks to his doctors and "nurses" for "protection" from life's adversities. The "regressed patient", seeking these qualities of "ideal parents" "in staff members" is disappointed by the absence of such qualities. "Thoughtful health professionals" "strive to enhance patients' feelings of "security" and "warmth" by helping make the environment (shared by both staff and patients) as "comfortable" and as "warm" as possible."

> Basic Nursing: A Psychophysiologic Approach, Sorenson Luckmann, W.B. Saunders Company, 1979, page 152

I need "chipper acting, cheery female nurses only" and "I need them all to give me hugs" and "rub my head to calm me down" and "hold my hand" through blood tests, shots, IVs, biopsies, or any other experiences involving sharp instruments just like I said in my first book I wrote about nurses comforting their patients.

"For some patients, e.g. patients in long term health care facilities, staff members become "pseudo-family members.""

> Basic Nursing: A Psychophysiologic Approach, Sorenson Luckmann, W.B. Saunders Company, 1979, page 152

These patients (and others) look to the staff for "protection", "warmth", "guidance", "support", "modeling", expectations and judgment they would hope to receive from their family. Security is enhanced for patients' expectations of them.

> Basic Nursing: A Psychophysiologic Approach, Sorenson Luckmann, W.B. Saunders Company, 1979, page 152

"It is thus desirable for health professionals to assess a patient's expectations of them and to identify ways in which these expectations can be dealt with constructively."

   Basic Nursing: A Psychophysiologic Approach, Sorenson
   Luckmann, W.B. Saunders Company, 1979, page 152

Like I said, some nurses I've run into in the past may think, "He acts like such a baby. Why do we have to deal with this? Why doesn't he just grow up? Do we have to baby him to death all the time and always do all these special things for him? Why do we have to be stuck with having to do this anyway?"

And, as you can see here, the answer is, "Well, you may feel that way, and like some have said, they feel like taking care of me is like having to take care of a kindergartner and they really don't like it, but if you really think about it, that's what you're there for because you are the nurses and you are the "mother surrogates" of all your patients.

This is especially true for disabled patients with special needs like my self and this is really what you need to do to make life better for both your patients and yourselves, and all goes better in the end when you do.

"Persons who receive their care from the same health practitioner are more compliant than those who are treated or examined by different practitioners. The explanation may be a combination of interpersonal "comfort", "ease of communication", and a "saving in time needed to explain problems".

   Comprehensive Rehabilitation Nursing, Nancy Martin,
   Nancye B. Holt, Dorothy Hicks, McGraw Hill Book
   Company, 1981, page 60

I do more for my nurse practitioner because she comforts me when I need her to and so does her daughter. She is very good to me, takes out time to listen to me, and advocates for me to others to help them understand my needs like she understands my needs.

"The brevity of the usual patient record also detracts from the ease with which another practitioner takes over. Problem-oriented records and flow sheets stating physical findings, lab tests, and medications or treatments are helpful in allowing a practitioner new to the case to grasp the whole picture. These records also assist the person's usual caregiver in following progress." "The relationship between the patient and the health practitioner" is one of the more important factors in compliance. This factor is difficult to measure, but that is probably not the reason few studies focus on it as a variable in compliance. The current emphasis on "patient characteristics" is a probable reason. Studies dealing with the relationship have examined it from the standpoint of patterns and content of communication on the part of the practitioner (usually the physician), "patient satisfaction with the encounter", "extent to which patient expectations are met", "amount of reciprocal interaction between patient and practitioner", and "congruity between what the patient thinks he or she is to do and what the practitioner thinks the patient is doing." In general, the studies have indicated that when the practitioner communicates in a formal, controlling manner, when there is little reciprocal interaction, and when patients' expectations are unmet, compliance is low."

> Comprehensive Rehabilitation Nursing, Nancy Martin, Nancye B. Holt, Dorothy Hicks, McGraw Hill Book Company, 1981, page 60

"There is an explicit time frame, a goal-directed approach, and a high expectation of confidentiality. The nurse establishes, directs, and takes responsibility for the interaction and the "client's needs" take priority over the "nurse's needs".

> Fundamentals of Nursing, 7th Edition, Potter and Perry, Mosby Elsevier, 2009, page 346

"In illness it should be expected that patients will regress to levels of behavior that are not as mature as those which they assume when well. They need to be allowed sufficient and appropriate "regression" and "dependence" in others."
>   Basic Nursing: A Psychophysiologic Approach, Sorenson
>   Luckman, W. B. Saunders Company, 1979, page 152

"Ill persons have a strong "need" for security, "warm", "friendly" interactions and familiar settings promote feelings of security."
>   Basic Nursing: A Psychophysiologic Approach,
>   Sorenson Luckmann, W.B. Saunders Company, 1979,
>   Page 15

"Nursing is a work of "intimacy". Nursing practice requires you to be in contact with clients not only physically but also emotionally, psychologically, and spiritually."
>   Fundamentals of Nursing, 7th Edition, Potter and Perry,
>   Mosby Elsevier, 2009, page 315

"In most other "intimate relationships", you choose to enter the relationship precisely because you anticipate that your values will be shared with the other person. But in the case of nursing, "you agree to provide care to your clients solely on the basis of their need for your services". Inevitably, "you will work with clients whose values differ from yours"."
>   Fundamentals of Nursing, 7th Edition, Potter and Perry,
>   Mosby Elsevier, 2009, page 315

"You will work with colleagues whose values differ from yours. To negotiate differences of opinion and value, it is important to have clarity about your own values: what you value, why, and how you respect your own values even as you try to respect those of others whose values differ from yours. A value is a personal belief about the worth of a given idea, attitude, custom, or object that sets standards that influence behavior."
>   Fundamentals of Nursing, 7th Edition, Potter and Perry,
>   Mosby Elsevier, 2009, page 315

"What behavioral qualities might patients find helpful in a nurse? Frequently people who are ill want to be "cared for" by a person who is "accepting", "thoughtful", "gentle", "nurturing", "kind", "genuine", "emotionally warm", "caring" and "giving".
> Basic Nursing: A Psychophysiologic Approach, Sorenson Luckmann, W. B. Saunders Company, 1979, page 132

"Professional nurses play a specific role in the management of health care. All clients in the health care system interact with a nurse at some point in ways that are unique to nursing. Nurses generally interact with clients over longer intervals of time than other disciplines. "Because nurses are often involved in "intimate physical acts" such as "bathing", "feeding", and "special procedures", clients and families reveal information not always shared with physicians, health care providers, or others."
> Fundamentals of Nursing, 7th Edition, Potter and Perry, Mosby Elsevier, 2009, page 319

"Details about family life, information about coping styles personal preferences, and details about fears and insecurities are likely to come out during the course of nursing interventions (Shannon, 1997)."
> Fundamentals of Nursing, 7th Edition, Potter and Perry, Mosby Elsevier, 2009, page 319

"Clients face situations that are "embarrassing", "frightening", and "painful". Whatever the feeling or symptom, clients look to nurses to provide comfort. "The use of "touch" is "one comforting approach" where "the nurse reaches out to clients to communicate concern and support".
> Fundamentals of Nursing, 7th Edition, Potter and Perry, page 101, Mosby Elsevier, 2009

"Touch" is "relational" and "leads to a connection between nurse and client". The skillful and "gentle performance" of a nursing procedure conveys "security" and a "sense of competence". "Caring touch" is a form of nonverbal communication, which successfully influences a client's "comfort" and "security", "enhances self-esteem", and "improves reality orientation" (Boyek and Watson, 1994). You express this in the way you "hold a client's hand", "give a back massage", "gently position a client", or "participate in a conversation".

> Fundamentals of Nursing, 7th Edition, Potter and Perry, page 101, Mosby Elsevier, 2009

"When using a "caring touch", the "nurse" is "making a connection with the client" and "showing acceptance of the individual."

> Fundamentals of Nursing, 7th Edition, Potter and Perry, page 101, Mosby Elsevier, 2009

"Patients" express frustration with the "impersonal" and "diffuse care" received in many large institutional settings. The nurse's focus should be on ensuring the "preservation of "personalism" and "continuity of care."

> Comprehensive Rehabilitation Nursing, Nancy Martin, Nancy B. Holt, Dorothy Hicks, McGraw Hill Book Company, 1981, page 569

"The nurse is responsible and accountable for individual nursing practice and determines the appropriate delegation of tasks consistent with the nurse's obligation to provide optimum client care. The nurse owes the same duties to self as to others, including the responsibility to preserve integrity and safety, to maintain competence, and to continue "personal" and "professional" growth."

> Fundamentals of Nursing, 7th Edition, Potter and Perry, Mosby Elsevier, 2009, page 315

"Compassion" asks us to go where it hurts, to enter into places of pain, to share in brokenness, fear confusion, and anguish. Compassion challenges us to "cry out with those in misery", "mourn with those who are lonely", "to weep with those in tears."
> Ethics in Nursing: The Caring Relationship, page 8,
> Veronica Tschudin, 2003

That's what I want in a nurse, "someone I can cry on when I am in distress and be able to receive their comfort". I also need "hugs" (be able to put my right ear on their cheek), and them to "rub the top of my head to calm me down" and "hold my hand" through needle sticks.

"Compassion" requires us to be "weak with the weak", "vulnerable with the vulnerable", and "powerless with the powerless". "Compassion" means "full immersion in the condition of being human."
> Ethics in Nursing: The Caring Relationship, page 8,
> Veronica Tschudin, 2003

"Nurses care when they are present with another with a "closeness" that evokes compassion. Hence the "caring nurse" is focused on the 'other' that the 'other's' welfare is paramount."
> Ethics in Nursing: The Caring Relationship, page 9,
> Veronica Tschudin, 2003

"Compassion is a complex aspect of caring. It demands above all knowledge of one's self and one's values."
> Ethics in Nursing: The Caring Relationship, page 10,
> Veronica Tschudin, 2003

"Compassion" is more specific than "caring". "Compassion" questions, brings to closure, and defends others. "Caring" calls for the caring; "compassion is there when it hurts." "Caring" can be professional, but "compassion has to be experienced."

> Ethics in Nursing: The Caring Relationship, page 10,
> Veronica Tschudin, 2003

"Caring can be learnt, but compassion comes out of the experience of one having been hurt and having been shown compassion. We do not respond to "compassion" out of a sense of duty but out of a sense of solidarity."

> Ethics in Nursing: The Caring Relationship, page 10,
> Veronica Tschudin, 2003

On page 11 of the book, "What Do They DO? Nurses" you will see a "friendly female nurse smiling and "holding a girl patient's hand".

> What Do They Do? Nurses, page 11, Jennifer Zeiger,
> Cherry Lane Publishing, 2010

On page 15 of the book, "What Do They Do? Nurses" you will notice a nurse "puts one hand behind the back of a male patient in a wheel chair" and "puts her other hand on his shoulder" and"looks at him" and "smiles".

> What Do They Do? Nurses, page 15, Jennifer Zeiger,
> Cherry Lane Publishing, 2010

The lady nurse on the cover of the book "What Do They Do? Nurses" is also "smiling cheerfully at a girl patient" as she takes her temperature.

> What Do They Do? Nurses, Jennifer Zeiger, Book Cover,
> July 2010

"Nursing is a profession that provides "care" to the sick, the injured and other people in need of medical assistance."

> World Book Encyclopedia Online, 2016

Once again, in the book "Clara Barton: Founder of the American Red Cross" you see "Clara "hold up a soldier laying down", "put her arm around him with one arm" and "give him a cup of water with the other hand" at the same time."

> Clara Barton: Founder of the American Red Cross, page 181, Augusta Stevenson, Aladdin Paperbacks, 1946 & 1962

In the Book, Clara Barton: Founder of the American Red Cross" it says this about Clara Barton. Clara's friend Susie got small pox and Clara took care of her and this was what was said about her:

"Mrs. White was grateful for all the help Clara gave. Clara seemed to know how to make her friend "comfortable". She could "soothe" her when no one else could."

> Clara Barton: Founder of the American Red Cross, page 143, Augusta Stevenson, Aladdin Paperbacks, 1946 & 1962

"That child is a natural-born nurse," said Mrs. White. "I don't know how I'd manage without her. What a wonderful help."

> Clara Barton: Founder of the American Red Cross, page 143, Augusta Stevenson, Aladdin Paperbacks, 1946, & 1962

"Clara Barton actually quit school for two years just to take care of him. He finally tried a clinic that promoted steam baths and other types of water cures and his health was restored in three weeks. If you will notice, "she puts her hand to his head" "holding a wet rag to her brother's head" while she "holds his arm with her other hand."

> "Clara Barton and Her Victory over Fear", page 15 Robert Quakenbush, Simon & Schuster Books for Young Readers, 1995

Now, you're probably going to say that's because it is her brother. In that case, get this, Clara went onto the battlefield to nurse people and nothing stopped her on her mission.

Clara had to dodge gunshots just to help the soldiers. Once "she stopped to give a fallen soldier a drink of water" and she "cradled him in her arms" but unfortunately a bullet passed under her arm hitting him and killed him.

"Clara Barton and Her Victory over Fear",
Robert Quakenbush, page 24 Simon & Schuster Books for
Young Readers, 1995

Speaking of a "compassionate nurse", look what I found in this book, "Gentle Annie: The True Story of a Civil War Nurse". Annie had men falling dead left and right off of horses "she tried to catch" while they were wounded and still alive.

Gentle Annie: The True Story of a Civil War Nurse,
Page 86, Mary Francis Shura, Scholastic Inc., 1991

"This is what the book says she did to the one she spoke to for a moment that then fell dead: "Blinking the tears from her eyes, she closed his gently. Then "she "touched" his cheek with the palm of her hand" "the way his own mother might have done if she had found him here."

Gentle Annie: The True Story of a Civil War Nurse,
Page 86, Mary Francis Shura, Scholastic Inc., 1991

Now that's comfort and compassion.

In the book, "Florence Nightingale–Demi" Florence Nightingale comments, "Nursing is one of the Fine Arts; I had almost said the finest of the Fine Arts."

Florence Nightingale, Una and the Lion, 1868
Florence Nightingale: Demi, Henry Holt and Company,
LLC. 2014

You will notice in the middle of this same book there is a page with a picture of a nurse "holding the hand" of a lady patient in bed and handing her a cup of water as well.

Florence Nightingale: Demi, Henry Holt and Company,
LLC, 2014

In the book, "Florence Nightingale: The Lady of the Lamp" it is stated that Florence Nightingale "paused many times bending down" to "place a cool hand" on a forehead or to "whisper soothing words."

> Florence Nightingale, The Lady of the Lamp by Kay Barnham, Raintree Steck-Vaughn Publishers, 2003

Now we are getting personal, but we're supposed to. We're nurses. We're the comfort providers, remember.

"Florence Nightingale considers herself to be a "mother" to her patients. She feels bad about leaving the men she took care of when she went home and left them in the Crimean grave. She makes the following comment concerning this, "Oh my poor men who endured so patiently. I feel I have been such a bad mother to you to come home and leave you lying in the Crimean grave. Seventy three percent from disease alone – who thinks of that now?"

> Florence Nightingale, The Lady and the Lamp, page 29
> Florence Nightingale, 1856 Kay Barnham, Raintree Steck-Vaughn Publishers, 2003

In the book, "Community Helpers- Nurses" you will notice on page 9 of this "non-fiction" kid's book "a lady nurse" is "bending over to "gently touch" a senior lady on the shoulder" that has a gas mask on as she lays in her patient bed "in the emergency room". They may have been putting this lady to sleep or giving her oxygen. This nurse "smiles sweetly" at her while she "touches" her shoulder and you can tell by the look in her eyes she cares for the lady and "wants to meet her needs and comfort her".

On page 21 of this same book, it says, "Patients are the first concern of nurses". Nurses are taught to see a patient's illness. They are also taught to 'see their feelings'. They want patients to be happy and healthy."

> Community Helpers: Nurses by Dee Ready, Ready Consultant: Marie Griffin, RN, C, Member of the American Nurses Association, Bridgestone Book, Capstone Press, 1997

In the book, "Nurses at Work" by Karen Latchana Kenney you will notice on page 25, it says that nurses need to be "caring" and "kind", and it shows a picture of a nurse "looking sweetly at a girl in bed" "with her hand on the girl's head", "on top of her hair even", not her forehead, even if she is taking her temperature.

I believe this lady is showing "comfort" to this girl "out of the goodness of her own heart" because "she is a compassionate nurse". And, this is a kid's book, yes, but it is a non-fiction kid's book about nurses so that facts found in this book are very real.

"Good nursing consists in securing as much "physical comfort" as possible for the patient in rendering prompt first aid in emergencies that may arise, and in "soothing" and "cheering" the patient's mind."

> Victor Robinson, Ph.C., M.D., Modern Home Physician, Wise, 1968

Even a doctor said nurses need to "comfort" their patients in this quote, and he said "physical comfort", but it's from 1968. Still, all the same, they still need to comfort their patients no matter when this quote was made.

"Nursing is also good preparation for raising a family. Nurses learn about health, illness, child care, and relationships among people."

> The New Book of Knowledge, N13, page 412, 1970

Like I said, you "treat your patients like children" and it "better equips you to take care of children and show them the compassion they need as well as your patients". It teaches you a lesson in how to "love" people, a very important lesson to learn in raising a family. You need to "care" for your patients not just see them as a number. You are their "caretaker" or "caregiver". Give them the care they need, don't just do your thing and send them away. "Comfort them". "Treat them like your own children".

To Nurse means to nurture. Nurture in the dictionary also means nourish.

I like a spelling thesaurus gadget a friend gave me. I don't really have trouble spelling. I just play with it for kicks to get meanings of words. According to this thesaurus gadget a friend at bingo gave me, the word nurse means "to act as a parent to." I've been looking for this definition the whole time. That's what I thought it meant.

So, you see, nurses are actually supposed to treat their patients as if they were their own children and provide the same love and affection toward their patients as they would their own child.

 To those who wish to be nurses, you are not just taking on a profession where you stick patients with a bunch of needles and help with surgeries and then receive a paycheck for it. "You are acting as a parent to these people."

"You are their caretaker and you are actually supposed to treat these people that are your patients like they are your children while they are under your care." "Anything you would do for your child from a "comforting" standpoint needs to be done for your patients." That's why I believe one of the people I copied the quote of in my book said that being a nurse is a great teaching tool for how to raise your kids. I think they meant that you were supposed to "comfort" them and "console them in their fear and pain" "with great compassion".

And, they did say in their quote that you are supposed to "comfort your patients", by the way. That means if they need you to "pat them on the shoulder", or "give them a hug", or "rub their head to calm them down and hold their hand" you need to do so. You have to do this for them. You would do this for your kids wouldn't you? Your patients need you to do the same for them no matter what their age. In case you think I am the only one emphasizing age one of the people I quoted said that "comfort should not be left to end of life care but that people of all ages should be comforted by their nurses."

So, you see, "nurses" were supposed to "comfort" their patients all along. It's just that some of the nurses in the bigger hospitals have let pride get in the way of their jobs as "comforters", and have stopped meeting their patients' needs, abandoning the earlier practices of nursing where "comfort" was the main key. Instead they think of themselves as someone above having to meet the needs of their patients, like they think they are business executives, when in fact, they are "caregivers" that are "responsible for meeting the needs of their patients", including "comforting" and "consoling" them in their fear and pain.

So, please remember to reevaluate your responsibility as a nurse and remember that comforting your patients is the key to good patient care.

By the way, one of your own medical professionals also made this quote almost exactly. I'm just confirming it. You didn't know I knew all this did you? Please make sure to remember to "comfort" me and all your patients when they come your way.

As I said, "any nurse" that is "unwilling" to "comfort" their patients" like a "mother would "comfort" her child or baby" "should not be a nurse" and "should find a different profession to work in".

"Patients worry about being treated impersonally. "A touch of the hand", "a stroke on the brow", "a look", "a pat", "the way a patient is handled", "made comfortable", and "helped" can all contribute to "making him feel valued and close to those caring for him."
> Basic Nursing, A Psychophysiologic Approach, Sorensen and Luckmann, W.B. Saunders Company 1979, page 159

"A patient is not truly "taken care of" unless the nurse helps him to feel, safe, secure, "loved", and as one who "belongs" rather than as an outsider who is viewed as in intruder"
> Basic Nursing, A Psychophysiologic Approach, Sorensen and Luckmann, W.B. Saunders Company, 1979, page 159

"The "well-being" of patients is of first importance to nurses. They take time to reassure worried patients and boost the patient's morale. Nurses are taught to recognize and understand "patients' needs" and provide emotional support as well as physical care."
> World Book, Number 14, N, page 617, 2006

You can see by reading this you need to encourage your patients and try to "cheer them up" and "be willing to "physically comfort them" "to make them feel better".

"To reinforce what I've already said about not needing an elaborate conversation with the patient, I suggest you try to remember a time when you yourself were really down and just prayed for someone who would understand. Chances are, you weren't looking for a lot of talk, but for someone who simply would listen and not be afraid to "touch" you."
> Dealing with Death and Dying, page 32, Nurseskillbook, Intermed, Inc., 1980

"If you can remember such a time, and most of us can, then you will know that you need to leave your "armor of professionalism" outside the door. Patients often feel repulsive, freaky, and unclean. "Touching" them, "putting a hand on their hand" or on the "nape of their neck" can mean so much, can make it a truly caring encounter."

> Dealing with Death and Dying, page 32, Nurseskillbook,
> Intermed, Inc., 1980

"If only we could be honest, both admit our fears and "touch" one another. If you really care, would you lose so much of your valuable professionalism if you cried with me? Just person to person? Then, it might not be hard to die…in a hospital…with friends close by."

> Dealing with Death and Dying, page 32, Nurseskillbook,
> Intermed Inc., 1980

Actually, this would make it easier to live for me, but only after continuously being this way with me when in a period of stress or grief.

I am already a very "touchy feely" person in the first place and need this kind of thing on a continual basis anyway, but I need it all the more during stress or grief, to a very great extent.

I also found this long account about how nurses are supposed to comfort patients treated in the ICU unit.

I have always been afraid I would be treated "impersonally" if I ever went to someone's "Intensive Care Unit (ICU)" but this is what this book, "Nursing Critically Ill Patients Confidently" has to say about the way "nurses treat their patients in the ICU ward".

"Although the ICU, by nature, doesn't allow privacy or dignity, do what you can to make the patient feel less like an object. Don't talk about him at his bedside, unless he is included in these conferences. Handle his personal belongings with extra care – these are the only things in the ICU he can call his own, so they take on special meaning for him. Taking the time to stop and talk, or even to just be near the patient is extremely important."

> Nursing the Critically Ill Patient, pages 30&32, Nursing Skillbook, Intermed Communications, Inc., 1979

"Touching" the patient's hand "gently" as you ask questions "can help show him that you care." Don't forget to introduce yourself before you "touch" a patient and "talk to him about the care as you give it", even if he's comatose or doesn't seem to respond. We've all probably had the experience of "caring" for a comatose patient, even of talking about him at his bedside, as if he didn't exist, only to have him tell us later exactly what had gone on around him. Try not to fall into this trap. Mr. Russell is not the "pneumonia on the ventilator" or a series of chest x-rays or blood-gas results. The complicated ICU gadgetry can distract you, but "resist the temptation of thinking of patients and treating them as objects connected to this machinery". "The best ICU nurse" "sees her patient first", "the patient's condition second", and "the equipment last."

> Nursing the Critically Ill Patient, pages 30&32, Nursing Skillbook, Intermed Communications, Inc., 1979

"If the patient can't talk but can communicate, give him a magic slate, an alphabet board, or a clipboard, paper, and pencil, and encourage him to use it. If possible, try phrasing questions to allow for a simple yes or no answer. Use every opportunity to observe the patient's mental status, as well as his physical condition."

> Nursing the Critically Ill Patient, pages 30&32, Nursing Skillbook, Intermed Communications, Inc., 1979

"If a patient seems depressed try to get him to think of the future rather than the not-very-pleasant present. Tell him when his family or friends call with a message and keep him aware of news and sports events- anything to get his mind off his illness."

> Nursing the Critically Ill Patient, pages 30&32, Nursing Skillbook, Intermed Communications, Inc., 1979

"If a patient acts too independent, he's probably frightened of the helplessness he feels. Try to include him in decision making and to avoid restraining him when possible."

> Nursing the Critically Ill Patient, pages 30&32, Nursing Skillbook, Intermed Communications, Inc., 1979

"Another patient may become totally "dependent" during illness and may look to an authority figure (like you) to solve all his problems." You may have to discourage this behavior once the patient's condition improves, but "it may be helpful to let him depend on you until then." Also try to be aware of how the patient interacts with family members. Remember, not all visits are beneficial, and destructive relationships can add to the patient's stress. If certain visitors seem to upset your patient, try to find out why and work with other members of the family to remedy the situation."

> Nursing the Critically Ill Patient, pages 30&32, Nursing Skillbook, Intermed Communications, Inc., 1979

I have always been a "dependent person" and have always been "dependent on others" with "dependency needs" and "need to be able to be "dependent" on my nurse" "when I am in the hospital setting".

"The emphasis on "comfort" and the role it plays in health care has changed in the last 10 decades. From 1900 to 1929, comfort was the central focus and moral imperative of nursing: from 1930 to 1959, "comfort" was considered a strategy for achieving fundamental requirements of nursing care: and from 1960 to 1980, comfort fell out of favor, to become only a minor aspect of nursing, and was significant only to people who received no medical treatment."

> Chia-Chia, Lin, PhD, RN
> School of Nursing, Taiwan
> Comfort: A Value Forgotten in Nursing-Lin, Chia-Chia
> PhD, RN Cancer, Nursing: November/December 2010-
> Volume 33- Issue 6-pp409-410

"During the last 3 decades, "comfort" has been relegated to end-of-life care where it is equated with the simplest aspects of care, which could be just as easily provided by nonprofessional caregivers." "Today, as always, "comfort" remains a substantive need throughout our "oncology nurses" play an important role in "promoting "comfort" through their lives.""Comfort is not a novel idea and has been cited by prestigious and cancer patients. In conclusion, comfort should not be relegated to end-of-life care. There is a powerful need for an increase in translational research to promote comfort in every stage of patient care. When "comfort" is emphasized in nursing care and "when promoting comfort becomes an important core value of nursing", I believe that "nurses will gain more respect from their patients", "the families of patients", and "our colleagues in the field of medicine."

> Chia-Chia, Lin, PhD, School of Nursing, Taiwan
> Comfort: A Value Forgotten in Nursing-Lin, Chia-Chia
> PhD, RN, Cancer, Nursing: November/December 2010-
> Volume 33, Issue 6-pp409-410

Please remember this when you take care of me. Thanks

Dear Nurses,

Please note my needs when you take care of me. I appear to be normal but I am actually autistic and have childlike needs. I need a lot of affection from cheery acting, chipper female nurses with motherly personalities who are caring and compassionate and willing to comfort me the way I ask them to comfort me. I have a sensory issue in my right ear that can only be relieved by putting my right ear on the cheek of the people I like, I call doing this a hug. So, I need to be able to do this with my nurses as well to bring me comfort, especially in medical situations, and I need to do it even worse when I'm scared. A cheery acting female nurse also needs to rub the top of my head and hold my hand to comfort me through an IV stick, blood test or shot, while another cheery acting female nurse does the stick. They also need to do this for me if I have a biopsy awake or have to be stuck with or cut with any other sharp instruments. It is really important I have these met. Those who have done this for me in the past did really well with me. I have a fear of needles and oversensitivity to pain. A shot and a blood test feel like being stuck with a steak knife. An IV feels like being stabbed with a butcher knife. A catheter feels like a sword being run through me. I need to be able to put Lidocaine/Prilocaine 2.5% cream on the site of the stick because of this. I need to be knocked out for all invasive procedures, as well as any catheter or tube insertions. I also need all the radiology techs and anesthesiologists and everybody that deals with me needs to be cheery, chipper acting females only and I need to be able to put my right ear on their cheek too because of my sensory issue. Male doctors, nurses, and techs tortured me as a child so I am scared of men. The serious trended female nurses also tortured me in childhood and adulthood so I am scared of them too. Please give me chipper acting, cheery female nurses to work with me only.

Dear Nurses,

For those of you who are unable to catch what all of my needs are on the letter you just saw who need to see them in list form, here is my list of needs again. Please meet all these needs on this list. Not doing so traumatizes me, so it's very important you meet these.

- Need All Chipper Acting, Cheerful Female Nurses Only
- No Male Nurses, Therapists, Techs, Radiologists, or Anesthesiologists
- No Serious Trended Female Nurses, Therapists, Techs, Radiologists, or Anesthesiologists
- Need Hugs from All My Nurses (A Hug to Me is Putting my Right Ear on Your Cheek)
- Need a Chipper Acting, Cheerful Female Nurse to Rub my Head to Calm me Down and Hold my Hand While Another Chipper Acting Female Nurse does the IV, Blood Test, or Shot
- They Also Need To Do This For Me If Any Biopsies are taken awake, or any Blades, Or Scalpels, or Other Sharp Instruments Are Used On Me Awake
- I Need to Be Able to Put on Lidocaine/Prilocaine 2.5% Cream on Site of Stick
One Hour Before A Needle Stick of Any Kind
- Need to Be Knocked Out For Any Catheter Insertions or Tube Insertions
(Heart or Urinary Catheter Insertions)
* Need to Be Able to Write Doctors/Nurses About Any Medical Conditions/Symptoms   I Have or Any Emotional Needs I Need Met
* Need All Medical Professionals Dealing With Me to Be Informed of the Needs
On this List and Be Willing to Meet Them

You meet this list and we are good to go. I still need to hug everyone I see so don't just limit it to one or two people that specifically work with me.

I need to be able to hug everybody I see when I go for a test in the Radiology Department for example, or the Pre-Op Department for example. Being able to do this helps me to be able to feel safe in my environment and comfortable with my nurses with the reassurance that anyone who does any other test on me in the same department will always be the same way with me as well as the ones that work with me, but do still only give me the chipper acting female nurses only to work with me because they are the nurses I am comfortable with. Plus, I have a sensory issue in my right ear that can only be relieved by being able to place my right ear on the cheek of all the people I like, including nurses. Not only that, but there are some tests that are so difficult for me to handle you may need extra assistance at times as well, so it is also better that everybody be prepared to give me a hug so I can feel at ease with everyone and know I will be taken care of in the way I need cared for with the comfort I need to receive from them in the way I need to receive it from them and not by what they decide but by how I tell them they need to comfort me, by giving me hugs, let me press my right ear on their cheek, and rub my head to calm me down and hold my hand through needle sticks. I need chipper acting cheery female nurses only to work with me.

The chipper acting cheery female nurses are the most compassionate people that do better at comforting me and making me feel at ease than anyone else. Male nurses and serious trended nurses tortured me as a child. Serious trended female nurses also tortured me as an adult. I need the chipper acting female nurses only to work with me that have cheery motherly personalities and comfort me the way I state I need comforted and I will be good to go. I am autistic and have childlike needs and need to be comforted in the way I ask to be comforted because this is the only thing that works for me. Please see to it that this is done for me, and we're set to go. Thank you.

Your friend,

Brian Gene Evans

To Read more about my life as a person with autism, be sure to read Autism Undiagnosed Part I – What Happened? , Autism Undiagnosed Part II- Will I Always Be An Outcast? And, Autism Undiagnosed Part III- Joys and Sorrows of Living with Adult Autism, a three part series by my wife, Bertha Marie Evans. Thank you. I hope you had a nice read and I hope this book gave you a better understanding of the needs I have that I need met by all my nurses in the medical field.

Also available are…

Victory: What Everybody Wants by Bertha Marie Evans

How to Have a Happy Marriage: Getting Past the Differences by Bertha Marie Evans

To schedule Bertha Marie to talk to your ladies church group or organization, contact her at (870) 416-1030.

She is an expert in adult autism, addiction, and abuse not only by study but by real life experience.

New Books Available by Brian Evans (or) Brian Gene Evans

"Big City Hospitals Don't Like Cowards"

"To Nurse Means to Nurture: The Need for Nurses to Comfort their Patients:

"To Nurse Means to Nurture Part 2: The Parent Role of the Nurse with All Ages of Patients"

"To Nurse Means to Nurture Part 3: Nurses Dealing with Patients with Anxiety Disorders

"Mainstreaming a Disabled Person into the Normal World is a Big Mistake"

"What Language Therapy Really Entails"

"Compassion for Disabled Peers in College is Needed"